CW00858440

BEAT THE DIET TRAP

Discover the truth about weight loss
and learn how to change
the habits of a lifetime

Janet Matthews Dip ION

September 2014

Copyright © 2014 Janet Matthews.

All rights reserved worldwide.

ISBN-13: 978-1505892130
ISBN-10: 1505892139

No part of this book may be reproduced by any means whatsoever without the written permission from the author, except brief portions quoted for the purpose of review.

This book is not intended to replace the services of physicians or other health professionals, nor as a substitute for the medical advice of medical or health professionals. The reader should regularly consult a physician in matters relating to his/her health and particularly with respect to any symptoms that may require diagnosis or medical attention.

Garamond font used with permission from Microsoft.

CONTENTS

❧❧

INTRODUCTION

❧❧

Do you feel you have been lied to by the weight loss industry?

Have you tried every diet going to no avail?

Are you confused by all the different weight loss plans available that contradict one another?

Do you exercise regularly and are still not able to lose weight?

Do you put off dieting because you really don't know what to eat?

Do you find yourself caught in **The Diet Trap**?

If you answered yes to any of these questions then join the club.

You may well have come across diet books that claim you can lose weight without dieting. While I agree that the majority of weight loss diets don't work, the idea of being able to lose weight without the need to change your dietary habits seems to me to be a contradiction in terms and immediately makes me feel as though I am being duped. According to Wikipedia, diet (nutrition) means the *sum of the foods consumed by an organization or a group*.

So with that in mind, we are all on a 'diet' whether we like it or not. What sets people apart however is the extent to which their 'diet' is healthy or unhealthy and whether they see their diet as a lifestyle choice or just a way to lose weight. I am sure the authors of these books are trying to move people away from fad diets, as well as using psychological tactics to help us to get over the 'diet hump', but it is important to accept that if we want to reach and maintain our optimum weight and be fit and healthy, we are going to need to make some dietary changes that we may find difficult. You are kidding yourself if you believe that eating low calorie Black Forest Gateau as part of your regime is the right way to go about losing weight and keeping it off. You need to be aware that there are some intrinsic reasons why you are overweight and why you find it difficult to lose that weight.

We are living in a time in history when there are more health clubs, more slimming clubs, more diet books for weight loss and more weight loss coaches than ever before, yet we have the highest number of overweight and obese people in the world. How did we manage to get to this stage? If we are following the advice available to us then surely we should all be slim, fit and healthy?

Sadly one of the reasons the latter isn't true is that we have been lied to. Basically the majority of weight loss diets don't work. The majority of exercise programs don't have the desired effect. One of the reasons is that many of them are too difficult to stick to, but also some of them are not telling us the whole truth. They are telling us many unfounded myths that are resulting in us misunderstanding the whole process of losing weight and maintaining our ideal body weight.

There are some basic questions that need to be asked. For example: Is it true that fat makes us fat? Does exercise really help us to lose weight without needing to change our eating habits? Can we really cheat the system and still lose weight, and more importantly keep it off? Or do these facts just make a lot of money for the food and fitness industry?

We are about to unearth some of the facts.

WHY I DECIDED
TO WRITE THIS BOOK

❧❧

Considering there are new diet and weight loss books being written and published on a daily basis, you may be wondering why I decided to write this book. Hasn't it all been written before?

I think the answer to that is both yes and no. Yes because much of it has been written before, but no because there always seems to be something missing or something not clearly explained. Sometimes there will be a weight loss myth or two lurking to confuse matters even more.

So my intention is simply to demystify weight loss by explaining what is happening in our bodies when we put weight on and why it can be so difficult to lose the weight and keep it off.

I have been involved with the health and weight loss industry for over 30 years. I have worked for two weight loss companies, run weight loss classes for a well known weight loss franchise and also helped numerous people to lose weight through personal coaching. Despite all of my experience I have never felt 100% comfortable with any of the well known weight loss regimes or the weight loss products used by the various companies I have worked for. They all felt very much like 'fad diets' that didn't teach the principles of a healthy lifestyle and an understanding of the importance of eating healthy 'real food'. They also failed to encourage each individual to discover what worked for them.

Since my teenage years I have probably been on just about every diet that has ever been produced (well almost). I have had some successes and I have had some failures. However I had never really cracked the code of what constituted a healthy successful weight loss diet. Every time I thought I understood what was happening, somebody moved the goal post and changed the rules and I was left in a state of confusion and skepticism regarding the whole weight loss industry. I am sure you will have had a similar experience.

So, in the midst of my confusion, I made a decision to do my own research into the truth behind the weight loss industry and ultimately the truth about what causes us to put on weight, why we find it difficult to lose it and how we can learn to lose weight easily and quickly and maintain that weight loss. If that is something you would like to learn, keep reading.

The obesity epidemic is at an all time high and the overweight population continues to grow. There has to be a more intrinsic reason why this is happening. Through my research I unearthed many weight loss myths but I also discovered some basic, scientific facts that I will be sharing in this book. These facts will be the key to beating the diet trap that so many of us find ourselves in.

You will discover:

- ➢ How the obesity epidemic first began.
- ➢ Why we gain weight (it's not what you have been told)
- ➢ The truth about the myths that surround weight loss.
- ➢ The truth about exercise, and its effect on weight loss.
- ➢ The link between obesity and degenerative disease.
- ➢ Tips and hints for managing a successful weight loss program.

And much more, so let's get started …

HOW OBESITY BECAME
A MODERN DAY EPIDEMIC

❧❧

Here are some disturbing facts about the overweight.

"More people are overweight than are under nourished."

*"Two thirds of British adults are overweight
and one in four is obese."*

*"The average person in Britain is nearly 3 stone heavier
than they were 50 years ago."*

There have been several suggestions as to why this might be. Every problem has a starting point and it may well be that the start of the obesity epidemic began in the 1970s when surplus corn was used to make High

Fructose Corn Syrup (HFCS), a sweetener that was cheaper, sweeter and more addictive than sugar. It also metabolizes to fat more rapidly than any other sugar

One of the first companies to use HFCS was Coca Cola and they were soon to be followed by many other popular brands. Today we find HFCS in a very large number of manufactured foods, including some foods that are sold as slimming foods.

Around the same time the era of the supersized portions was born, and diners in America were serving mammoth sized breakfasts and other meals and snacks encouraging their clients to eat more and more food.

The combination of HFCS and the supersized meals were to play a big part in contributing to the obesity crisis that was hitting first America and then the UK and now many other countries in the world, especially those who have adopted a western diet.

THE TRUTH ABOUT THE
WEIGHT LOSS INDUSTRY

∞∾

HOW AMERICA DISCOVERED IT HAD A WEIGHT PROBLEM

Louis Dublin, a statistician at the Metropolitan Life Insurance Company in the United States, looked into the statistics regarding the correlation between early death and being overweight. In order to increase the premiums charged to the customers he made the body weight acceptable for cheaper policies lower than it needed to be. This classification meant that more people were deemed to be overweight.

As a result, the insurance company made more money from the inflated policies but, more importantly, the US government took these statistics onboard. As a result of this arbitrary decision by Louis Dublin, America believed it had a weight problem and the weight loss industry was born.

THE RISE OF THE WEIGHT LOSS INDUSTRY

Despite the fact that the weight loss industry was offering advice and diet products to the overweight population, the majority of them were still struggling to lose weight. It soon became evident that WEIGHT LOSS DIETS DON'T WORK. But this was even greater fuel for the weight loss industry as the success of their business relied on the fact that people didn't lose weight and so came back for more. The dieters blamed themselves rather than the product for the lack of weight loss. If they did blame the product they would then search for another method of losing weight. The newest fad diet craze was always there to give them renewed hope.

Over the years there have been many weight loss crazes from slimming meals in a drink to weekly weight loss clubs like Weight Watchers and Slimming World. Whatever the craze might be the bottom line is that the weight loss industry only makes money when people fail to lose weight and return for more of the same.

Dr Carl Henegan, director for evidence based medicine at Oxford University claims that over a 5 year period weight loss groups such as Weight Watchers are not effective in helping people to lose weight and maintain their weight loss. He found that only 20% had maintained their weight after 2 years and just 16% after 5 years.

The success of Weight Watchers and other similar companies relies on the fact that 85% come back in the future and try again.(As quoted by the CEO of a well known weight loss company)

Soon after companies like Weight Watchers became successful they were taken over by the big food giants. Heinz bought Weight Watchers in 1978 followed by Slim Fast(a protein meal replacement drink)which was bought by Unilever in 2000 and Jenny Craig which was bought by Nestle. Before too long weight loss foods were appearing in our supermarkets, enticing people to buy with the promise of losing weight.

The supermarkets are a walking paradox. In one aisle you will find all the processed and packaged foods that contribute to making us fat and in another aisle you will find the low fat, low carb, so called 'healthy' slimming products that aim to help us lose weight but in fact are keeping us fat. It is a sad fact that a large number of people are on a perpetual diet.

To illustrate the hypocrisy of the food industry, I have checked the ingredients of several of these so called healthy options diet foods.

Here is one as an example:

Reconstituted Dehydrated Potato (50%, Water, Potato Flake, Preservative - Sodium Metabisulphite), Water, Lamb (11%), Onions, Carrots, Concentrated Tomato Puree, Peas, Diced Tomatoes (Tomatoes, Tomato Juice, Salt, Firming Agent - Calcium Chloride), Modified Tapioca Starch, Worcester Sauce Barley Malt Vinegar, Water, Treacle, Soya Sauce (Water, Soya Beans, Wheat, Salt), Brown Sugar, Salt, Lemon Juice, Color - Plain Caramel, Anchovy Paste (from Fish), Glucose-Fructose Syrup, Oil of Cloves, Tamarind, Garlic Extract, Chilli Pepper, Spirit Vinegar), Salt, Beef Stock (Beef Stock, Water, Maltodextrin, Salt, Vegetable Fat, Vegetable Concentrates (Carrot, Celery, Celeriac, Onion), Tomato Concentrate, Chicory Fiber, Yeast Extract, Glucose Syrup, Sugar, Herb and Spice Extracts, Spice), Yeast Extract (contains Barley), Flavorings (contain Milk, Smoke Flavoring), Color - Plain Caramel, Cream Powder (Cream Solids, Skimmed Milk Powder), Parsley, Mint, Black Pepper.

As you can see there is glucose syrup and glucose - fructose syrup, brown sugar and maltodextrine listed in the ingredients. Although maltodextrine isn't exactly a sugar it has a high GI of 105 and therefore converts rapidly to glucose increasing the blood sugar response in the blood.

WHY DO WE PUT ON WEIGHT IN THE FIRST PLACE?

❦

We have already discovered a couple of the reasons why obesity has become an epidemic. The introduction of HFCS and the introduction of supersized meals has had a major impact, but this doesn't address all of the reasons why we have an obesity problem.

We need to look at why some people are obese and others aren't. Why does HFCS and supersize factor in some people's diet and not in others. It is important for each of us to ascertain why we put weight on so that we can address the problem and successfully deal with it.

A Lack of Knowledge

The majority of our eating habits are formed in our early years, primarily in the home. My own children grew up in the 1970's when the obesity epidemic was starting to emerge. I remember being given advice from the health visitor regarding how to feed my children. We were advised to start mixed feeding at 6 weeks (I believe it is now nearer to six months). There was an array of baby foods to choose from along with a well known brand of rusks and other wheat based products. There seemed to be no knowledge of appropriate foods to feed a 6 week old baby or even how much to give them. The rule was simply if they are hungry then feed them.

As a result my daughter, who was my first born, was overweight by the time she was one year old and I had to make a decision to put her on a diet before the weight became a permanent fixture. She was a hungry baby who loved her food and so I fed her accordingly. I am horrified now when I look back and can't believe how much things have changed for the better.

There is so much information available today and so much more encouragement regarding feeding babies the right foods at the right time and not starting mixed feeding too soon. For some reason my maternal intuition kicked in before it was too late and as a result of the dietary changes I made, my daughter started to lose some of her excess weight and returned to an acceptable weight for her age and height.

Parents today receive far better education regarding feeding their babies, and there is so much more information on the internet for parents who want to go one step further and give their children the very best start in life

All education regarding healthy eating doesn't happen in the home, although that is where the habits are formed. School also plays an important part in health education, both regarding the food they serve to the pupils at lunchtime and the education they provide the pupils regarding why and how to follow a healthy diet. Unfortunately many schools serve poor quality, high carbohydrate meals, often to enable the suppliers to stick to a limited budget.

Healthy eating is often taught as a subject through Health Education but it needs to be carried through at school meals times in order for it to be taken on board by the pupils, otherwise it becomes theory without the practice and this will often be instantly forgotten. Unfortunately education has been through some times of change in the last twenty years and not always for the better. As a result Home Economics took a backward step.

I was trained as a Home Economics teacher back in the 70's (commonly known as Domestic Science in the UK) when cookery was taught throughout the school and pupils were encouraged to prepare healthy well balanced meals. In the UK when Home Economics became part of Design and Technology, the emphasis seemed to change from planning healthy meals to planning the design for the box to put biscuits in. I am being a little facetious here but the emphasis changed and cookery, as I knew it, seemed to disappear from the curriculum.

As a result we are now seeing a generation many of whom do not have the cookery skills required to prepare wholesome home cooked meals for themselves and their families. It is unlikely that any noticeable improvements will be able to be made with that particular generation but hopefully if our current cohort of pupils are taught about healthy eating and cooking real food, the tide will begin to slowly turn.

EMOTIONAL EATING

I am sure that most of us can identify with the concept of emotional eating. When we suffer emotional problems many of us eat for comfort. If those emotional problems are short lived then often the emotional eating stops and life reverts to normal and no harm is done.

If, however, the emotional problem is deep rooted and more chronic in nature, then the emotional eating is going to continue until the cause of the emotion is dealt with.

Emotional triggers might include:

> *Feeling sad or depressed.* This can result in us eating to raise our spirits.

> *Boredom or loneliness.* How often do we find ourselves eating to fill that emptiness? It gives us something to do and helps us to feel better, but only in the short term.

> *Social cues.* The regular mid morning cream cake or pastry with colleagues or coffee and biscuits with a friend becomes a habit that is very difficult to refuse.

> *Advertising.* An advert for a particular treat can easily persuade us to buy when we are feeling low and in need of a pick-me-up.

All of these triggers will result in some sort of emotional eating and depending on your own personal situation the triggers can have either a small or a big effect on your eating habits and subsequently your weight.

A lot of emotional eating is due to learned habits. We associate feeling better with having a cream cake or eating a tub of ice cream. It is a little bit like drinking alcohol or smoking, the habits are formed and we become aware that the habit helps us to feel better. Breaking these habits can sometimes be an effective way of dealing with this problem, but of course it can take a lot of will power, something we don't always have enough of when we are feeling down. As a matter of interest it takes a month to break a habit and 3 months to re-establish a new habit.

If the emotional problem is deep seated then it may be necessary to talk to a counselor or to find a therapist who practices The Emotional Freedom Technique (EFT) to see if they can help you deal with the root of the emotion you are struggling with:

http:// www.emofree.com/eft/

Discovering how to deal with emotional eating is enough for a book on its own. I am simply mentioning it here as a trigger for over eating or eating the wrong foods

STRESS

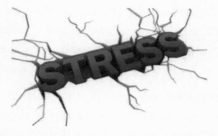

Stress has a similar effect to our emotional problems. When we are stressed we are less likely to eat a hearty salad and more likely to choose a bar of chocolate or a sugary treat. Somehow the sugary treat seems to hit the spot and helps us to 'feel' better in the short term.

I remember when I was teaching, we would have a staff meeting once a week and as a treat we would bring home made cakes and biscuits like flapjacks and brownies. It was our treat to ourselves after a stressful day. Inevitably one treat would turn into two or three treats. After all we had worked hard and deserved it !!

It is worth being aware that stress not only causes emotional eating, but also the release of cortisol and adrenalin, which can affect the metabolism by slowing it down. It can also encourage fat storage. So stress has a two pronged attack on your weight loss success.

Again this is beyond the scope of this book but some ideas for dealing with stress might include:

- Meditation.
- Yoga.
- Exercise.
- Cutting back on commitments.
- Relaxation.
- Aromatherapy massage.
- Finding time to have fun with friends and family.

Ideally you need to look at the root cause of your stress and find ways to eliminate it rather than managing it with the techniques listed above, but they are a good starting point if stress is currently one of your problems.

If you are interested in learning more about what causes stress and how to deal with it, my book *Is Stress Your Silent Killer?* is available on Amazon.

INSULIN RESISTANCE

Insulin resistance is not only the cause of weight gain but is probably the number 1 factor that prevents you from successfully losing weight and keeping it off, so understanding what it is and what to do about it is very important if you are serious about losing weight.

When you eat a meal, the carbohydrate content is broken down by the digestive system and it is converted into glucose, which then circulates in the blood stream so that it can be used by the cells in your body for energy.

The hormone insulin is responsible for storing any excess glucose that isn't utilized by the body. If you are insulin sensitive then you will only need a small amount of insulin to store glucose.

Every time you eat foods containing carbohydrates more insulin is released to deal with the excess glucose. Because there is a limit to the amount of glucose your body can store insulin stores it as fat.

If your diet has been high in carbohydrates and processed foods your body will become resistant to insulin and every time you eat more carbohydrate more insulin is produced.

High insulin levels means more fat is stored, but not only that, high insulin levels also means fat can't be released from the cells, and so it is harder for the body to lose weight.

So you can see how this can very easily become a vicious circle that has to be broken in order for weight loss to take place. Luckily dealing with insulin resistance is relatively straight forward.

I am sure you have already guessed from the information above that the best cure for insulin resistance is to drastically cut down on the carbohydrates and processed foods that cause a blood sugar spike, and increase the amount of protein and fresh vegetables in your diet.

Proteins are able to slow down the absorption of carbohydrates (sugar) which in turn helps to lower the amount of insulin required.

Exercise is also an important factor in the management of insulin. Exercise decreases the body's requirement for insulin by lowering the amount of sugar in the blood.

SET POINT AND THE YOYO EFFECT

Research that has been done with animals and humans has discovered that each person has a programmed 'set point' weight.

According to Dr Michael T Murray, one of the world's leading authorities on natural medicine:

"The 'set point' is the weight that a body tries to maintain by regulating caloric intake. It has been postulated that individual fat cells control this set point: when the fat cell becomes smaller, it sends a powerful message to the brain to eat. Since the obese individual often has both more and larger fat cells, the result is an overpowering urge to eat.

The existence of this set point explains why most diets don't work. While the obese individual can fight off the impulse to eat for a time, eventually the signal becomes too strong to ignore. The result is rebound overeating with individuals often exceeding their previous weight. In addition, their set point is now set at a higher level making it even more difficult to lose weight. This effect has been termed the 'ratchet effect' and 'yo-yo' dieting."

It would appear that the set point is intrinsically linked to the degree of sensitivity of the fat cells to insulin. So as we have seen, insulin resistance is evident in the overweight individual due to an over consumption of

BEAT THE DIET TRAP

carbohydrates. We can now add the 'set point' to our vicious circle, demonstrating even more the problems the overweight population may have losing weight and maintaining that weight loss

We are what we eat AND digest - so looking at digestion and why poor digestion may be causing the weight problem is also an important factor.

Very often on any weight loss diet, there will be a period of time when the weight seems to plateau. At this point the body feels it is at its normal weight and so sticks happily to that weight despite the fact that you are still following the same diet.

If this happens then it is time to change what you are doing. Maybe you need to add some more exercise, particularly high intensity exercise and strength training (more on that later). Increase your protein intake or cut down on a few more high GI carbs. It may be a case of trial and error to see what your body responds to. With so many things it is just a matter of listening to your body to find out what works best

ALLERGIES

Allergies to certain foods such as wheat and gluten are thought to be the cause of unexplained weight gain and difficulty in losing weight

According to Dr John Mansfield, a leading pioneer in the field of allergy and nutrition:

> *"Food sensitivities are by far the most common cause of weight gain rather than too many calories or lack of exercise."*

Dr Mansfield identified the 20 foods most likely to produce a reaction, starting with the most common:

- Wheat
- Corn
- Milk and products made from it
- Corn (maize)
- Eggs
- Yeast (used in many products such as bread, vinegar and alcohol)
- Cane sugar
- Coffee
- Oats
- Barley (malt)
- Beet sugar
- Tea
- Potatoes
- Soy (used frequently in processed foods)
- Lemons
- Cocoa beans (chocolate)

- Oranges
- Beef
- Pork
- Onions

Mark Hyman MD, an expert in functional medicine, believes that food allergies can lead to weight gain and can also be the reason why you find it difficult to lose weight. According to Dr Hyman food allergies cause inflammation in the gut and inflammation is known to cause insulin resistance. As we have already discussed insulin resistance results in the body producing larger amounts of insulin and insulin is a hormone that stores fat, mainly around the belly. It is therefore very important to ascertain whether or not you have allergies that may be hindering your ability to lose weight.

Depending on where you live you may be able to ask your doctor to do a blood test to ascertain if you have any allergies, otherwise you will need to pay privately. Once you know what your allergies are then you can eliminate them and see if that makes any difference to your weight loss. Again it is a matter of listening to your body and being more aware of the effect of certain foods.

If you are unable to afford to have tests done a cheaper option might be to book an appointment with a kinesiologist who will be able to ascertain what your allergies are through muscle testing. Alternatively you can do an elimination diet where you eliminate the possible allergy forming foods for a couple of weeks preferably one at a time and then reintroduce them and make a note of the effect.

Five years ago I found out that I had a gluten sensitivity. I discovered that gluten had damaged the lining of my gut causing leaky gut syndrome. This in turn was allowing undigested particles of food to be in contact with my immune system. This in turn was causing inflammation as well as increasing insulin resistance.

As we have already discussed, insulin is the main reason for weight gain and ultimately obesity. When I eliminated gluten from my diet I found that my body naturally returned to my ideal weight without the need for any further dieting. As with all dietary changes there were times when this was difficult for me to stick to and I soon realized to my cost that not eliminating gluten meant that I was inclined to put on weight.

A leaky gut can be caused by many things. Allergies are just one of the causes, but it may be simply down to a bad diet. A diet high in processed foods, sugar and low fiber foods will feed the bad bacteria in the gut upsetting the ecosystem. Inflammation soon follows and undigested food particles and toxins are absorbed into your bloodstream. This can lead to fatty liver and increased insulin resistance.

Remember, too much insulin in the system is what causes us to store fat. It also causes us to be more prone to disease and, due to its ability to limit the lifespan of our cells; it leads to more rapid aging.

What more reasons do we need to discover if we have hidden allergies that are causing our health problems?

If you feel that you have a gluten allergy/intolerance or leaky gut syndrome, you can find more information in my book *Really Healthy Gluten Free Living*.

Myths Surrounding Weight Loss

❧❧

There are many myths surrounding weight loss that have actually been the cause not only of preventing people from losing weight, but have actually been responsible for them gaining weight in the first place.

Fat Makes You Fat

That is certainly a statement that would seem to make sense. Many people believe that the fat we eat is the fat that covers our bodies. However all may not be as it seems. Fat is in fact an integral part of every single cell in our bodies. It is required for the digestion and absorption of the fat soluble vitamins (A, D, E and K),as well as being required to access dietary protein.

Fat is also a source of energy. There are also certain essential fats that are required for the management of inflammation.

Fats are an *essential* part of our diet and avoiding those means they cannot perform the vital roles necessary to keep our bodies healthy.

However if we eat too much fat will the body then store it as fat?

Not necessarily.

Fats in themselves do not make us fat.

They do not mobilize insulin like sugar does but they do have the ability to **satisfy the appetite**. Sugar, on the other hand, does not satiate and it does mobilize the insulin.

I addition, the sugar spike, followed by the sugar, low results in you feeling hungrier sooner, and subsequently craving even more sugar.

Unfortunately the low fat lobby, which started in the 1970's, has been unhelpful to those with coronary heart disease. Individuals with weight problems have also been consuming these unhealthy low fat products that, more often than not, have added sugar to improve the taste.

A cardiologist in the UK has recently spoken out in favor of turning the tide on saturated fat and is recommending a high fat low carbohydrate diet. An article reporting on the subject in the Daily Mail[1] states:

> *"The assumption has been made that increased fat in the bloodstream is caused by increased saturated fat in the diet ... modern scientific evidence is proving that refined carbohydrates and sugar in particular are actually the culprits."*
>
> Professor David Haslam,
> National Obesity Forum

If we look even further back than the 1970's we will find the following experiment demonstrating the beneficial effects of a high fat diet on weight loss:

> *One of the earliest obesity experiments, published in the Lancet in 1956, comparing groups on diets of 90 per cent fat versus 90 per cent protein versus 90 per cent carbohydrate revealed the greatest weight loss was among those eating the most fat.*
>
> Daily Mail Online October 24th, 2013

---

[1] http://www.dailymail.co.uk/health/article-2472672/Is-high-fat-diet-GOOD-heart-Doctors-say-carbs-damaging-arteries.html

WE NEED TO EAT LESS AND EXERCISE MORE

This is another statement that on the face of it would seem to make sense but in this case the opposite is actually the truth. We need to eat more and exercise less. This doesn't seem to make a lot of sense until we look further into the meaning behind the words.

Eating More

If you cut down on the amount of food you eat it can have several negative effects regarding your ability to lose weight.

- Firstly you will find that you feel hungry and dissatisfied and are more likely to suffer from cravings which could well result in your eating more of the wrong type of foods to satisfy your cravings.

- Secondly if you consume too few calories you body has to make a choice, either it loses fat or it loses muscle and guess what, your body chooses to lose lean muscle.

Consuming regular well balanced nourishing meals ensures that your energy levels are consistent. Eat when you are hungry and eat until you feel full, as long, of course, as you are eating real wholefoods. This also ensures that your blood sugar levels and insulin levels are regulated which, as a result, serves to reduce cravings.

BOTTOM LINE:

Eat more of the right foods

Exercise Less

In a recent study at the University of Copenhagen a group of men doing exercises for 30 mins a day lost 7 lb on average after 13 weeks. A second group of men exercised for 60mins, and lost just 5 pounds after 14 weeks.

Although this doesn't prove anything conclusively, the answer seems to lie in more efficient exercising. High Intensity Interval Training (HIIT) has been found to be an efficient exercise for weight loss and takes no more than 20 -30 mins if done correctly. However if you want a toned body then short bursts of strength training, 10 - 20 minutes, 3 times a week is probably all that you need.

One of the reasons that exercise becomes the 'big baddy' is that exercising for an hour or more a day 5 days a week is unrealistic for the majority of people (unless you are addicted to your fitness regime) and the result is that you will do it for a few weeks and then you will give up.

If you can manage to do the HIIT and the strength training, then all the better. If not then you need to choose whether strength and toning are top of your list or turning your body into a fat burner.

You will find more information on the correct exercise for weight loss in a future chapter

IT DOESN'T MATTER WHAT YOU EAT AS LONG AS YOU RESTRICT YOUR CALORIES

The American Paradox

A study called 'Divergent trends in obesity and fat intake patterns : The American Paradox' by Adrian F Heini was reported in The American Journal of Medicine in 1997.

The study observed that between 1980 and 1990 the American population reduced their calorific intake and their fat intake by 4% and 11 % respectively. In addition the consumption of fat free foods rose from 19% to 76%. Despite all of this, obesity rose by 31% during the same period. Needless to say those carrying out the study found these facts difficult to comprehend and had no choice but to conclude that there was no correlation between calorific intake and weight gain.

There are so many misconceptions regarding calories. If you believe that too many calories will cause you to gain weight, you might also be of the opinion that all you need to do to lose weight is to reduce your calorific intake. *'Calories in equal calories out'* is a popular catch phrase.

As we can see from the study above, this is not strictly true. For a start 'all calories are not created equal'. You could eat 3 slices of fruit cake and consume 1000 calories or you could have salmon and salad and a sugar free apple crumble and probably consume no more than 600 calories. Which one do you think your body would respond most favorably to?

You need to be aware of a few truths here:

1. It is sugar that makes you fat not calories

This is a phrase I will be reiterating throughout the book in the hope that it is the message you will take away with you.

Fat is stored as a triglyceride. Triglycerides are formed from 3 fatty acids that are bound together by glycerol. By providing the body with more glucose more glycerol is made, resulting in more triglycerides being made and more fat being stored in the fat cells. Remember that glucose is made from the breakdown of carbohydrates during digestion.

2. Simply restricting calorific intake does not guarantee weight loss

Serious calorie restriction has been practiced successfully for years, in particular, as a way to promote anti aging and longevity. The group of people who engage in this practice are called CRONies and they follow the CRON-diet (Calorie Restricted with Optimum Nutrition).

However just restricting calories without any thought regarding the nutritional value of the calories you are consuming isn't the answer, whether it is for longevity or for weight loss.

The calories must come from nourishing home cooked food, not from processed or ready meals. It certainly shouldn't come from foods high in carbohydrates, especially foods with a high glycemic index (more on that later) as they convert more readily into glucose and subsequently into fat.

Restricting the amount we eat and increasing the amount of exercise we do makes the incorrect assumption that the body is able to burn stored fat. Most of us have become carbohydrate burners, which means that the body will always use carbohydrate for fuel first. The body will only burn fat when there is no glucose/glycogen available. Modern man rarely, if ever, allows his body to get to the state where it can burn its own fat – let alone will.

However, there is a specific regime that encourages the body to be a fat burner, it is called Intermittent Fasting. I will be explaining how this works in a future chapter.

FAD DIETS AND FAST WEIGHT LOSS ARE THE BEST WAY TO GO

Please believe me, **fad diets don't work**.

By fad diets I am referring to diets that promise fast weight loss and generally rely on a few specific foods, for example the cabbage soup diet or the grapefruit diet. The main reason they don't work is that they are short term diets and they do nothing to help you to change your eating habits for the long term. Short term gain is about all they can offer. They are generally so restrictive that they are almost impossible to stick to for any length of time. Any 'diet' that is going to work has to be a lifestyle change not just so you can lose weight for a special event but for life.

Many of these diets offer fast weight loss but very often the weight loss in the first week is primarily loss of fluid and the second weeks may well be loss of muscle due to the fact that the diet doesn't include sufficient protein and other vital nutrients. And guess what? When you start eating your normal diet again you put the weight straight back on. This is prime example of short term gain.

Over the years I have tried numerous fad diets in a desperate bid to lose weight before a big occasion, I have done the grapefruit diet, one with a concoction of orange juice and raw eggs, high protein diets, meal replacements, restrictive calorie counting, and many others that I have now forgotten. All of them worked for a short while, but none of them taught me how to change my dietary habits, eat healthily, and keep the weight off.

ARTIFICIAL SWEETENERS ARE A GOOD LOW CALORIE REPLACEMENT FOR SUGAR

For years the belief has been that artificial sweeteners were beneficial for anyone on a weight loss diet, after all they had so few calories and they enabled us to have our sweet craving satisfied. It is no surprise that we are now discovering that artificial sweeteners are not as beneficial as they were once thought to be.

Apart from a long list of possible health hazards (here is a link to a list of studies from 1970 to the present day:

http://aspartame.mercola.com/sites/ aspartame/studies.aspx

Artificial sweeteners such as aspartame can actually cause you to gain weight. This is mainly due to the fact that aspartame increases insulin sensitivity, and as we discussed earlier we know that insulin sensitivity results in the body storing fat and not easily letting go of it.

Another interesting phenomenon here is the fact that when we eat something sweet that contains sugar, as well as your body releasing the pleasure neurotransmitter dopamine it also releases a hormone called leptin. Leptin has the job of informing your body that you have had the required number of calories, an indication that you are full.

If you have foods sweetened with an artificial sweetener the brain still releases dopamine but it doesn't activate leptin so the body is left feeling hungry. As a result you will undoubtedly end up consuming more calories before the appetite regulating hormone leptin kicks in and your appetite has been satiated.

DISEASES THAT ARE
LINKED TO OBESITY

❧❧

There are a number of overweight people who are keen to promote and celebrate their size rather than do anything about it. While I am in favor of everyone having the freedom of choice to do what they wish, and while I also applaud the positive attitude of those who are happy with their size, I do have concerns about the potential for disease in overweight and obese individuals. There are several diseases that have been linked to obesity.

Rather than seeing obesity as being the 'cause' of these diseases it might be more accurate to view it from the point of view that the eating habits that have lead to obesity are the same eating habits that have caused the various diseases.

If the food you are eating has resulted in you being overweight or obese the chances are you are eating the wrong sort of food, and that food will also have a detrimental effect on your health.

Diseases that are linked to obesity include:

- Coronary heart disease.
- Cancer.
- Type 2 diabetes.
- High Blood Pressure.
- Osteoarthritis.
- Gall Bladder Disease.
- Gout.
- Asthma.
- Sleep Apnea.
- Fatty Liver Disease.

So even if you are quite happy with your size, you certainly shouldn't be happy with your dietary habits and the long term effect they may be having on your health.

It is generally accepted that most diseases are caused by inflammation in one or other area of the body.

The foods that cause inflammation are as follows:

- Sugar and foods containing sugar raise blood glucose levels. This in turn causes the release of cytokines, chemical messengers responsible for the body's inflammatory response

- Foods containing gluten and other allergens. The body has an inflammatory response when these foods are ingested

- Trans fats (hydrogenated fats) and other fats that may cause free radical damage also cause an inflammatory response. These would include certain margarines, foods such as cakes and biscuits prepared with hydrogenated fats) and cooking with polyunsaturated fats such as sunflower oil.

Eliminating any food that can cause an inflammatory response will lessen your chances of a degenerative disease as well as being a healthier diet that will aid your weight loss or prevent you from gaining weight in the first place.

How A Healthy Attitude Can Help You To Lose Weight

⋘⋙

The best way to lose weight and keep it off is to ensure that you include the following in your weight loss regime:

- You must change your attitude towards your weight loss. (More on this in the **Bonus** included at the end of the book)

- You must consider health first and weight loss second. If you are not healthy you won't lose weight.

- You must change your dietary habits.

- You must eat real food as nature intended.

- You must eliminate sugar from your diet.
- You must include the right sort of exercise in your daily regime.

Two approaches I have found to be very successful for weight loss are Intermittent Fasting and choosing foods according to their Glycemic Load. Both of these work well independently but together they are a formidable combination

INTERMITTENT FASTING

What is Intermittent Fasting?

The general understanding of fasting is going without food for a day or more at a time. Friday was always accepted as a fast day by the early church, and many spiritual practices include fasting as a regular part of their practice.

Intermittent fasting is slightly different. Rather than fasting for a whole day and going without food completely it is only necessary to go without food for a certain amount of time, or as the name suggests going without food intermittently. Historically we have accepted our sleeping hours as a time of fasting and typically break that fast in the morning when we have our breakfast (break fast) . Intermittent fasting is a little more regimented than the random over night fast, as some people may eat at 10 pm and have breakfast at 7 am which only gives the body 9 hours of fasting. With intermittent fasting, the optimum time for fasting is around 16 - 18 hours. So if you had your evening meal at 6 pm you would not eat again until around 12 noon the following day. You would then eat your normal diet between the hours of 12 noon and 6 pm.

The above regime could be practiced every day, in which case the normal amount of daily calories would be consumed between the hours of 12 noon and 6pm.

Alternatively you can fast on two days and eat normally at other times. This has become popular way to lose weight and is known as the 5:2 diet. On the days that you fast you must limit your calories to 500 for woman and 600 for men. This would appear to be the regime of choice for those wanting to lose weight and can, if preferred be practiced over three days instead of two and would then become alternate day fasting

Intermittent fasting is beneficial because it give the body a time without food to enable regeneration

I can personally vouch for this method of losing weight. Due to a small weight gain after my summer holidays I decided to follow the 5:2 diet, with restricted calories on the fasting days. I lost about 7lb quite easily in a few weeks. Several members of my family did the same diet and had similar results. It was the easiest diet I have ever embarked on and at no time did I feel hungry. I also noticed that on the day following the fast I didn't feel inclined to eat more than normal to make up for the lean day. Other benefits we experienced included steady energy levels, no food cravings and improved sleep.

My daughter, who had weight to lose after the birth of her fourth child, has kept up the IF for the majority of the last 12 months, taking time away from it only during the holidays. She has steadily lost weight over that time and has never struggled to keep to her diet

HOW DOES INTERMITTENT FASTING WORK?

Intermittent Fasting has been attributed to both the body's ability to lose weight and also to the increase in longevity. So how does this work for:

a) *Weight Loss*

As I mentioned in an earlier chapter, for the body to burn fat it needs to be in fat burning mode. The biggest difficulty that dieters experience is that most of the time our insulin levels are high as a result of the food we are eating.

Insulin will remain high for some time but will drop once your body has digested and absorbed the food you have recently eaten. This is the fasting stage and the best time for your body to burn fat while your insulin levels are low. This is why IF works so well because during the extended fasting periods your body is in fat burning mode

b) Increasing Longevity

The fact that IF increases longevity is certainly a bonus for anyone using IF to lose weight. The theory behind this assertion seems to hinge on something called Insulin-like Growth Factor(IGF1).

IGF1 is responsible for the division and production of new cells, however when the levels of IGF1 fall below a certain level the body stops producing new cells and starts to repair old ones instead. It is possible to repair DNA damage and can even protect us from age related diseases.

In a study with rats done way back in 1945 by A J Carlson and F Hoelzel, showed that: "Apparent life span was increased by intermittent fasting."In their summary they stated:

> *The optimum amount of fasting appeared to be fasting 1 day in 3 and this increased the life span of littermate males about 20% and littermate females about 15%.*
>
> http://jn.nutrition.org/content/31/3/363.full.pdf

JANET MATTHEWS

A study done by James Johnson, Donald R Laub and Sujit John in 2003 came to a similar conclusion:

> ***Restricting caloric intake to 60–70% of normal adult weight maintenance requirement prolongs lifespan 30–50% and confers near perfect health across a broad range of species.***
>
> http://www.medical-hypotheses.com/article/S0306-9877(06)00089-2/abstract

By administering alternate day fasting, consuming 20 - 50% of the normal daily intake on the fasting day and normal eating on the other day, they discovered health benefits occurred by the end of the first 2 weeks. Improvements in conditions such as insulin resistance and auto immune diseases and many other degenerative diseases were observed.

A more recent study by Krista A Varady and Marc K Hellerstein, reported by the American Society for Clinical Nutrition in 2007, reviewed human and animal trials on the affect of alternate day fasting and chronic disease. Although they summarized that ADF had positive effects on both cardiovascular disease and cancer, they concluded that:

> *ADF may effectively modulate metabolic and functional risk factors, thereby preventing or delaying the future occurrence of common chronic diseases, at least in animal models.*
>
> *The effect of ADF on chronic disease risk in normal-weight human subjects remains unclear, however, as do the mechanisms of action.*
>
> *Much work remains to be done to understand this dietary strategy fully.*
>
> http://ajcn.nutrition.org/content/86/1/7.full

Does IF cause the body to go into starvation mode and a lowered metabolism? Starvation mode dates back to the years when food was in short supply in times of famine, when humans were required to adapt so that they didn't starve to death.

During these extended periods of starvation the body lowers its metabolic rate(the rate at which we burn calories) enabling it to survive until the next food appears.

With regards to IF and starvation mode, one study showed that the body's metabolic rate lowered after 60 hours of fasting:

http://www.ncbi.nlm.nih.gov/pubmed/3661473

So it would be unlikely that IF would affect the metabolic rate as the hours of fasting are generally no more than 18 hours.

With regards to concerns about loss of muscle mass, it would be worth considering eating plenty of protein prior to and following your fast so that the muscles have plenty to feed on. Apparently it is only in prolonged fasting that protein catabolism becomes a problem.

If amino acids are in short supply due to lack of food then the body uses the protein from the muscles. The amino acids are then converted into glucose so that blood glucose is maintained. With IF this will not be an issue as the fasting periods are generally too short

THE GLYCEMIC LOAD

One of the most important things to remember on any diet is *you are what you eat*. Choosing healthy natural food is a vital part of a healthy diet and especially one that promotes weight loss. Consuming foods that have a low Glycemic Load (GL) can be very beneficial in any weight loss regime. However we need to understand the Glycemic Index, the precursor to the Glycemic Load, first.

What is the Glycemic Index?

The Glycemic Index is a way of measuring the effect that different carbohydrate foods have on our blood sugar levels.

All carbohydrates do not have the same metabolic response. Typically foods that raise blood sugar are high on the GI scale and foods that are low on the GI scale provoke a low blood sugar response. As we have learned earlier sugar is not helpful for anyone trying to lose weight. It raises the level of insulin in the body and insulin keeps the fat in the fat cells.

It is therefore sensible to choose foods that are low on the GI scale. The recommendation is to choose foods below 55; any foods with a GI of 55 or above should be avoided or eaten very occasionally with protein to lessen the glycemic load.

The following chart (courtesy of Wikihow cc) shows the high GI foods that are best avoided and the low GI foods that are best to include in your diet.

High Glycemic Index (>55)	Low Glycemic Index (<55)
White bread Pumpernickel bread Pita bread (white)	Barley bread 100% whole wheat bread Corn tortilla Wheat tortilla
Soft drinks Gatorade	Unsweetened apple juice Unsweetened orange juice Tomato juice
Cornflakes Instant oatmeal	Bran cereal Old-fashioned oats
Couscous White rice	Pearled barley Quinoa Brown rice Bulgur
Regular ice cream	Milk Reduced-fat yogurt
Banana Grapes Raisins Watermelon Russet potatoes Sweet potato Beets	Apple Grapefruit Orange Peach Pear Black beans Chickpeas Lentils Cashews Peanuts Peas Carrots
Pretzels	Hummus

Obviously the lower the GI the less the blood sugar response will be and the smaller amount of insulin will be needed to deal with the sugar spike.

The first person to pioneer the Glycemic Index for weight loss in the 1980's was a Frenchman called Michel Montignac. **The Montignac Method** was not considered to be a diet but rather a lifestyle and a new way of thinking about weight control. Montignac considered dieting to be limiting the amount of food we eat. The Montignac Method is not about eating less but about eating more of the right foods. It is about making informed choices. You can read more about The Montignac Method and see his comprehensive list of foods and their GI on his website:

http://www.montignac.com/en/
the-montignac-method/

What is the difference between the Glycemic Index (GI) and the Glycemic Load (GL)?

More recently in addition to the Glycemic Index (GI) we now have another measurement called the Glycemic Load (GL)

Whereas the GI ranks a carbohydrate according to how quickly it raises your blood sugar levels, the GL measures how much it will raise it? GL is based on the GI of the food multiplied by the amount of carbohydrate in the food divided by 100. For example a food that has a GI of 60 and contains 5g of carbohydrate has a GL of 5 x 60 / 100 = 3

Because some foods may have a high GI but a low carbohydrate content the GL is seen to be a more accurate measure. You will be pleased to know that there is no need for you to remember this formula as there are GL charts available to help you quickly identify the GL of the food you want to eat.

For a comprehensive GL chart you can visit

http://naturalnutrition.uk.com/glycemic.pdf

According to Patrick Holford in his book *Burn Fat Fast, The alternate day low GL diet plan*, there are several ways you can lower the GL of your meal:

- Combine protein with carbohydrate.

- Include foods that contain high levels of soluble fiber such as oats and chia seeds.

- Add lemon juice or vinegar. This slows down gastric emptying, which lowers the Glycemic Load.

Patrick also suggests that you eat no more than 40 GLs a day and that you divide that into 10 GLs for each main meal plus 5 GLs for snacks mid morning and mid afternoon.

DOES EXERCISE HELP WEIGHT LOSS?

❧❧

Over the years there have been many differing opinions regarding the effect of exercise on weight loss.

As far back as the 1950's, a study of obese children was conducted by Jean Mayer, the director of the School of Nutrition at the Harvard School of Public Health. It was observed that some girls took part in activities such as ballet and cheer-leading, however none of the obese children being observed took part in these activities.

As a result an incorrect assumption was made that children are obese because they don't exercise rather than concluding that the more overweight a child becomes the less active they become.

More recently Professor Terry Wilkins did a similar research study which spanned over 11 years. Professor Wilkins also discovered that a child who is overweight is less likely to want to do exercise, however, despite this observation, he concluded that more exercise did not lead to weight loss, but that weight loss depended on the food that we eat.

Many people are getting the wrong message regarding exercise. The food giants have exacerbated the situation by promoting the message that it is ok to eat their 'less than healthy' products provided you do plenty of exercise.

Fitness clubs and gyms have promoted the benefits of cardio and the need to burn the excess calories. Wilkins is of the opinion that the majority of us (of which I am definitely one) will not be able to sustain the amount of daily cardio necessary to lose weight. Nobody is saying that cardio is useless, just that it requires supreme effort and determination to keep up the regime. Remember we are talking about weight loss here and not any other benefits that cardio might have.

I mentioned earlier that it is all about doing more efficient exercise. It is the old adage 'you need to work smarter not harder'.

HIGH INTENSITY INTERVAL TRAINING

High Intensity Training requires that you use maximum effort in a quick burst of energy to achieve muscle fatigue and the maximum use of oxygen. If done correctly your body will continue to use high amounts of oxygen several hours after the training has finished and burn calories for up to 48 hours after.

The "interval" part of the training requires alternating periods of high intensity exercise followed by periods of low intensity exercise.

By combining these two types of exercise you are essentially maximizing aerobic and anaerobic fitness, as well as maximizing fat burning and muscle building. The other benefit of course is that your workouts will be shorter. Studies have demonstrated that 27 mins of HIIT three times a week has the same benefit as 60 mins of cardio five times a week. There really is no contest.

However HIIT can be very demanding and needs to be approached according to your current level of fitness. An appropriate regime that is suitable for you should be followed for both effectiveness and safety.

There is an excellent infographic that explains the system admirably on this site:

http://greatist.com/fitness/complete-guide-interval-training-infographic

HIIT need only be done two or three times a week. On the other days you can alternate between resistance training, core exercises and stretching. This will ensure a good all round exercise regime.

STRENGTH TRAINING

Strength training is one of the most effective ways of burning fat. It is important for health and improves bone density. You don't need any fancy equipment, just your own body weight and exercises such as squats, pull ups and press ups. Simply pushing and pulling your own weight.

CORE EXERCISES

Your core muscles are located in your abdomen, your back and your pelvis. There are 29 in total and all of them need to be exercised in order that you can protect and strengthen your back. They enable you to have good posture and protect you from unnecessary injury. Exercise regimes such as Yoga and Pilates are excellent for strengthening the core muscles. Most areas have local classes that you can join to ensure that you are doing the exercises correctly

STRETCHING

Stretching improves circulation and helps to increase the elasticity of muscle joints. Yoga is also excellent for incorporating stretching into your regime.

The above information is purely to make you aware of the different type of exercises that need to be performed

I am not qualified to give advice regarding the specific exercises suitable for you, so I would suggest that if you want to take these exercises seriously, you need to find a trainer to help you devise a personal program or a purchase a program that you can follow that has been written by a qualified fitness coach.

For those of you who really struggle with exercise, the Human Performance Institute have recently demonstrated that you can fulfill the requirements for a high intensity workout using just your own body weight, a chair, and a wall

This animated video on Dr Mercola's site shows you a 7 minute exercise routine that fulfills these requirements.

**http://fitness.mercola.com/sites/fitness/
archive/2013/05/24/7-minute-workout.aspx**

There is also a pdf of the exercises if you prefer a hard copy to refer to. It is important to do the exercises in the correct order (as shown on the pdf) to ensure that opposing muscle groups have the chance to alternate between working and resting

http://i.dailymail.co.uk/i/pix/2013/05/10/article-2322470-19B6EE7F000005DC-949_634x380.jpg

Tips To Help You To Get The Most Out Of Your Weight Loss Regime

❧❧

Law of Attraction

I was undecided as to whether I should include this, mainly because so many people get the wrong idea about it. They have the misguided notion that you can attract what you want simply by dreaming about it and thinking about it all day long. Of course this is nonsense. The Law of Attraction only works when you take action and allow it to take its course. It does however take a positive mindset. There is no use starting a diet with the belief that it won't work or that it is too hard to stick to, or you don't like this food or that food.

The Law of Attraction requires that you imagine yourself to be slim, behave as if you are slim and that you are taking action to achieve your goal and believe that what you are doing will reap rewards. It is also important to ensure that you have chosen a diet that has all the right attributes. It must be a healthy diet that you wouldn't mind sticking to for the rest of your life and is full of healthy nourishing real food. No processed or commercial weight loss foods, just plain old healthy food as nature intended. Of course you can prepare the food in an interesting and appetizing way but your meals must be made from fresh food that you will prepare and cook yourself.

It might be helpful to find a photograph of yourself before you put weight on and that can be the image you keep in your mind's eye to help you to set your goal.

REMOVE TEMPTATION

I know from my own dieting attempts that it is vitally important to remove temptation. This can be very difficult if you are living with others who are not on the same healthy weight loss program. However you should try to impress upon them that you need their support and even if they don't want to lose weight your new healthy eating regime would also be beneficial for them if only to improve their health.

By transforming your store cupboard and removing foods that you shouldn't be eating you are helping yourself to stick to the diet. You may see it as a waste of food but it would also be a waste for you to spoil your diet by eating it. It goes without saying that the same applies to the food you buy. Only purchase healthy fresh foods that are synonymous with your new way of eating.

TRANSFORM YOUR STORE CUPBOARD

In order to successfully transform your store cupboard you need to understand what you are looking for. Here is a list of foods you may or may not realize are not good for your health and are certainly not good for your weight loss diet.

1. Sugar, white or brown- an obvious one I know - but one of the first foods you need to eliminate from your diet for all the reasons we have already discussed.

2. All foods that contain sugar and other sweeteners either HFCS or artificial sweeteners.

3. Any processed or packaged foods that contain anything other than the basic food ingredients.

4. Low fat foods even if they have no added sugar.

5. Polyunsaturated fats (liquid at room temperature) especially those that have been hydrogenated to make trans fats (one of the most dangerous fats for your health).

6. White flour and white flour products such as bread and pastries.

Here also is a list of foods you should be including in your store cupboard:

1. Lots of fresh low GL fruit and vegetables.
2. Good quality meat, grass fed, free range and organic if possible.
3. Fish, both white and oily, from sustainable and unpolluted sources
4. Pastured eggs (free range).
5. Nuts and seeds.
6. Good quality fats and oils such as coconut oil (this oil can actually help you to lose weight).
7. Superfoods such as avocados, chia seeds and goji berries

With all of the foods you should be eating you need to check on the GL and make sure the total number per day is kept to 40

KEEP A WEIGHT LOSS JOURNAL

The findings of a yearlong study were published in the *Journal of the Academy of Nutrition and Dietetics*. The study discovered that keeping a weight loss journal was the number 1 tip for weight loss success. Those who kept a weight loss journal lost consistently 6lb more than those who didn't keep a journal. The reason given was that they were more likely to hold themselves accountable for the food they ate.

The author of the study, Dr Anne McTiernan commented that:

> *"It is difficult to make changes to your diet when you are not paying attention to what you are eating."*

One of the most important things to remember is that self deception will always end in failure. If you want to succeed then keeping a weight loss journal will encourage you to be honest and discourage you from giving in to temptation. It will also be a good indication of whether your diet is working and whether you need to make some tweaks

You need to record absolutely everything you eat and everything you drink. Everything counts. You may also want to record how much you exercise. This may include your exercise sessions and any sports you may play. It may also include a shopping day when you seemed to walk around the shops for hours on end or day when you spent several hours digging in the garden, or decorating the bedroom. An accurate record will give you a full picture of your week and help to explain why you lost or gained the weight you did when you weigh yourself at the end of the week.

If you have lost weight at the end of the week then you will know that the foods you ate and the exercise you did were sufficient to ensure success. If you didn't lose weight or worse still you gained weight then you know that your regime didn't work and changes are necessary for the following week. You can't do this if you don't keep accurate records of everything you eat and drink

Henry Ford said:

> ***If you do what you've always done,
> you'll get what you've always got.***

If your previous dietary habits didn't have the desired effect, you need to make some changes.

WEIGH AND MEASURE YOURSELF AT THE START OF YOUR DIET AND TAKE 'BEFORE' PHOTOS.

Most people think about weighing themselves but many will not think to take measurements. I remember going on a diet some years ago just before my daughter's wedding. I weighed myself after a couple of weeks of starting the diet and I was really disappointed with my lack of weight loss. I then measured myself and was shocked at the amount of size I had lost. When you are dieting correctly you will lose fat and gain lean muscle and of course muscle weighs heavier than fat so what doesn't show on the scales will often show on the tape measure.

Taking "before and after" photos seems to have gained popularity in the last few years. The most effective photos are taken in the same place with possibly the same or a similar outfit (in some cases a bikini or swimming shorts if you are brave enough)

One cautionary note is not to be tempted to weigh or measure more often than once a week as weight can fluctuate daily and it is easy to be disheartened. It is however, important to weigh at the same time of day in the same clothes, on the same scales in exactly the same place. There is always a discrepancy according to the time of day, and scales placed on a tiled floor as opposed to a carpet or a rug will always weigh differently.

PLAN YOUR MEALS IN ADVANCE

Depending on how organized you are it is a good idea to plan your meals in advance. There is nothing worse than getting to meal times with no idea about what you are going to eat. These are the times you are most likely to cheat and have something quick and easy that isn't a part of your diet food.

Some people like to plan a week's meals in advance and then they can purchase the foods they will need to prepare those meals. Others may prefer just to think of a day at a time. But whatever you do make sure you have plenty of healthy food available to choose from.

From my own experience I have discovered that if I don't plan at least a few days in advance I can easily end up either not having the ingredients I need or wasting food that I have bought and not used. Neither of these is to be advised.

INFORM YOUR FRIENDS AND FAMILY THAT YOU ARE ON A DIET AND ASK THEM TO SUPPORT YOU

There is nothing worse than being motivated to start a diet only to find that friends and family don't fully support you. I don't mean that they literally don't support you, but their actions can be less than helpful. The friend who brings you a cream cake because she feels sorry for you and thinks you are being deprived, or the family member who makes comments about you not eating enough.

These things can easily weaken your resolve and it is during these times that you either need to have the strength to stand up for yourself or you can decide to give in on that occasion. If you decide on the latter it is important that you're not too hard on yourself and also that you don't feel downhearted that you have broken your diet. One cream cake once in a while is unlikely to do any harm (so long as it doesn't become a habit) Just get back to your diet as soon as possible.

The reality is that most people will not keep to a diet 100% of the time and you should allow yourself a meal a week or maybe even a day occasionally when you are officially off your diet. This way you will avoid feeling deprived and be more likely to stick to your new regime the remainder of the time. We all get invited out for a meal or to a party and the last thing you want is to feel miserable because you can't enjoy the food. Just enjoy yourself without going over the top and get back to your diet as soon as possible.

MAKE THE CHANGES SLOWLY IF NECESSARY

Depending on your previous eating habits it may be beneficial to make your dietary changes over a period of time. If you had a diet made up of mainly convenience foods and lots of bread, pastries and sweet foods you may not feel able to make the change overnight. Cutting out sugar would be the most important change - but even then you may want to cut down gradually over a few weeks.

You must keep in mind that this is NOT a weight loss diet. It isn't just about losing weight; it is a diet for life. It is a life changing decision to change your eating habits. You need to be ready to make that commitment. I am sure that you will find it much easier than you think. The real food diet is much more satisfying than any other diet.

Of course there will be some people who need to make the changes in one go; an all or nothing approach. This may require a little more willpower but may also be a way of getting rid of your old eating habits and starting a new regime. Everybody is different and part of this process is about understanding yourself and listening to your body.It is more empowering if you take responsibility for the choices you make and then you are more likely to follow through with them and stick to them.

ROME WASN'T BUILT IN A DAY

That may be true but it was built one step at a time and that is what you have to allow yourself the time to do. Remember, if we want to change a habit we need to repeat it for 30 consecutive days for it to become a new habit. Some people even believe it can be done in less than 30 days.

The same goes for dieting. Take your time and remember this is a diet for life; it is not just a diet to lose weight. You need to establish a new habit, a new way of eating and a new way of viewing your health and well being.

Remember, you have to be healthy to lose weight. If you concentrate your efforts on eating a healthy well balanced diet your weight loss will be an automatic outcome.

It is my opinion that you can't successfully lose old habits and create new ones if you just 'think' you would like to change your habits. There needs to be a deeper change of heart, a deeper understanding of why you are making a change. In the case of weight loss you need a real desire to have a healthier lifestyle and an acceptance that the old ways are a thing of the past.

Motivation is the most important part of having a successful outcome.

I would like to share an experience I had recently regarding my own motivation to finish this book.. During a coaching session, finishing my book was one of my goals. I was asked how motivated I was to finish my book. I said 8 out of 10. I was then asked what it would take to make that 10/10. I said I didn't know if I could make it 10/10. My coach then challenged me to think about my reasons for writing the book. Why was I doing it? As soon as I became aware of my "why" my motivation soared to 10/10

The same applies to a healthy diet. You need to be very clear why you are doing it and your reasons need to be very solid.

Ask yourself what your motivation is to lose weight and be healthy. If it isn't 10/10 then you need to work hard to get it to 10/10 if you want to be successful

REFERENCES

❧❧

Here is a list of references I have used for my research and links that I have referred to in the book that I think would make interesting further reading.

Links:

http://www.dailymail.co.uk/health/article-2472672/Is-high-fat-diet-GOOD-heart-Doctors-say-carbs-damaging-arteries.html

http:// www.emofree.com/eft/

http://www.nationalobesityforum.org.uk/http://aspartame.mercola.com/sites/aspartame/studies.aspx

http://jn.nutrition.org/content/31/3/363.full.pdf

http://www.medical-hypotheses.com/article/S0306-9877(06)00089-2/abstract

http://ajcn.nutrition.org/content/86/1/7.full

http://www.ncbi.nlm.nih.gov/pubmed/3661473

http://www.montignac.com/en/the-montignac-method/

http://naturalnutrition.uk.com/glycemic.pdf

http://greatist.com/fitness/complete-guide-interval-training-infographic

http://fitness.mercola.com/sites/fitness/archive/2013/05/24/7-minute-workout.aspx

http://i.dailymail.co.uk/i/pix/2013/05/10/article-2322470-19B6EE7F000005DC-949_634x380.jpg

Books I recommend

Burn Fat Fast: The alternate-day low-GL diet plan by Patrick Holford and Kate Staples

ABOUT THE AUTHOR

❧❧

Janet Matthews lives in Hereford in the UK with her husband and has 3 children and 4 grandchildren. She is a retired head-teacher of a centre for pupils with emotional and behavioral problems.

Janet completed a diploma (Dip ION) in nutritional practice from the Institute of Optimum Nutrition in London in 1988 and has had an active interest in health and personal development for many years.

Her other qualifications include:-

> * Life Coaching Diploma.
>
> * Enneagram Teacher (part 1).
>
> * MBTI Practitioner.
>
> * Metabolic Typing Practitioner.

Janet has been writing online as a ghostwriter for over 6 years and has several health related blogs of her own. She has also been a guest writer for other blogs and websites on the subject of health and well- being.

You can visit her website for updated information on her books, products and recommendations.

http://your-healthy-options.com

You can contact her via email

janet@your-healthy-options.com

Or alternatively visit her author page

http://www.amazon.com/Janet-Matthews/e/B009L1FVNK/

If you liked this book and feel you have benefitted from the information you have learned, please take a moment to write a review on Amazon. Reviews go a long way to helping me reach others and share this material.

Thanks for your support.

Janet Matthews

OTHER BOOKS BY JANET MATTHEWS

<u>REALLY HEALTHY GLUTEN FREE LIVING</u>

How to heal your gut with a healthy gluten free diet - includes 32 healthy gluten free recipes

Synopsis

If you have Celiac Disease or Gluten Intolerance and want to know how to live a healthy gluten free life, and where to find gluten free recipes that will help to heal your gut and put you on the road to recovery, then this is the book for you.

There is a tendency to think that just because you are on a gluten free diet that all your problems will melt away. If you suffer from Celiac Disease or a Gluten Intolerance then removing gluten from your diet is certainly the first step towards improving your health and well being but it is far from the whole story.

Gluten can have a devastating effect on our bodies, so much so that we can experience numerous symptoms that just won't completely go away whatever we do. The bottom line is that we are impairing our immunity and need to redress the balance before we succumb to more serious diseases and health problems in the future. 80% of our immune system is in the gut and we can't afford to ignore gut related problems if we are to live long and healthy lives

In Healthy Gluten Free Living you will find the answers you have been looking for. As well as an explanation of why gluten causes damage to the gut, you will also discover which foods are safe to eat and which foods are capable of healing the damage to the gut.

Finding suitable gluten free foods and gluten free recipes is half of the battle, the other half is knowing how to use them wisely to improve your chances of recovery.

There are many gluten free recipe books available, but it is important to be discerning about the ingredients used in these recipes. Gluten free doesn't always equal healthy gluten free. This requires knowledge and understanding

In Healthy Gluten Free Living you will find healthy gluten free recipes that are aimed at healing the damaged gut and allowing the body to heal itself.

In this book you will discover:-

- What gluten is and what foods you will find it in
- What to do when you have been diagnosed with Celiac Disease or Gluten Intolerance
- How to eliminate gluten from the diet
- Whether all gluten free foods are healthy alternatives
- What causes leaky gut
- How to heal a leaky gut
- The difference between gluten free and grain free
- Lots of healthy healing gluten free recipes
- Resources to help you learn more about healthy gluten free living

Having suffered from gluten intolerance myself I have firsthand experience of how to approach a healthy gluten free diet and lifestyle. My personal experience in addition to my professional experience has provided me with the resources to offer the information you will find in this book, to my readers.

What others have said

A fantastic book for anyone looking to turn their health around and embrace a gluten free lifestyle. Inside you'll find lots of great gluten free recipes, tips and tricks to getting gluten free and staying that way. The author also shows lots of gluten free mistakes beginners make when selecting the true gluten free products. It's one book you'll return to many many times on your path to better health.

Sean White (amazon.co.uk)

I was so pleased to find this book. I am gluten intolerant and have gradually removed gluten from my diet, but so many of the gluten free foods are just junk. This book is a breath of fresh air as it explains how you can be gluten free and also heal your gut and eat a much healthier diet.

I have tried several of the recipes and was really impressed, (raspberry and banana ice-cream yum yum) and will be adding a couple more to my diet on a regular basis soon.

If you suffer digestive complaints, bloating or lethargy get this book and try gluten free, you may be pleasantly surprised.

Book Lover (Amazon)

IS STRESS YOUR SILENT KILLER?

*HOW TO DEAL WITH STRESS AND ACHIEVE
PERMANENT STRESS RELIEF*

A dramatic title for a topic that is so often glossed over. Stress is responsible for many of today's diseases and illnesses. Stress and anxiety compromises your immune system and your body's ability to absorb the nutrients from your food. But is stress relief enough to prevent Illness and disease invading your body or do we need to change our way of thinking and being in order to learn how to deal with stress before it starts?

Most people will have encountered one or more episode of stress in their lives and in many cases with sensible stress management techniques, will have learned how to deal with it and will have suffered no long term ill effects. But what happens if you have many episodes of protracted stress in your life and your body is unable to cope with the constant rush of adrenalin into the blood stream? Stress relief is far more difficult to achieve when you are suffering from chronic stress. It is also time maybe to reassess your life, and discover what is really causing you to be stressed. You may be surprised!

Chronic stress such as this can lead to serious health problems if it is allowed to continue and can all too easily become YOUR Silent Killer. This short book can help you to recognize the symptoms and help you identify appropriate strategies for how to deal with stress and ultimately enjoy stress free living.

Having suffered from chronic stress myself, I am only too aware of the detrimental effect this can have on our health and well-being. In this book I will share my own experience, what it taught me about myself, and how, through a deeper inner knowledge, I was ultimately able to begin to stress proof my life.

In this book you will discover

- What Stress is
- The signs indicating my own stress
- The main causal factors of stress
- Main causal factors of my own stress
- How stress leads to ill health
- How stress affects the immune system
- Strategies for dealing with stress
- What I discovered in hindsight
- How I alleviated my stress
- My long journey back to spiritual, emotional and physical well-being

Through my journey you will learn not only how to achieve stress relief but how to deal with stress by gradually eliminating it from your life. Stress free living is possible once you know what it is about YOU that makes you stressed. Very often it isn't simply the circumstances of our busy lives that makes us stressed, but something more intrinsic in the way we think.

What others have said

The author Janet Matthews describes her book as "a short book with 13,334 words." A HUGE book of 13,334 words would be a more apt description. Every word, concept and verbal illustration carries tremendous weight and meaning that I, for one, can recognize, identify with, and use to my benefit.

Julia Busch – AntiAgingPress.org

What is really good about this book is the connection the author makes with the reader through her own experience which will help many people understand that they are not alone in their situations. Even if you feel you are coping with stress this book will help not just deal with it but combat it.
Is Stress Your Silent Killer? - worth the investment.

Liam Lusk

MEDICAL DISCLAIMER

THE CONTENTS OF THIS BOOK ARE provided for informational and educational purposes only. They are not intended to be a substitute for professional medical advice, diagnosis, treatment (including medical treatment), psychotherapy, counseling, or mental health services.

Consult a physician or other qualified health professional regarding any opinions, information or recommendations with respect to any symptoms or medical condition.

The information and opinions expressed in this publication are believed to be accurate and sound, based on the information available to the author.

BONUS

꘎꘎꘎

THE SEVEN HABITS OF HEALTHY PEOPLE (FOR HEALTHY WEIGHT LOSS)

Steven R Covey's book *The 7 Habits of Highly Effective People*, was the inspiration for this booklet. On his website it says:

> *The 7 Habits of Highly Effective People* has been a top seller for the simple reason that it ignores trends, and pop psychology for proven principles of fairness, integrity, honesty and human dignity.

Using the principles in Steven Covey's book I would like to outline an approach that will help you to live a healthier and happier life and will also help you normalize your weight and help you to understand why you need to eat in a particular way to maintain your health and your weight

HABIT 1: BE PROACTIVE

Being proactive is about taking responsibility for your life and the choices you make. If you are proactive you accept that your life is your responsibility and you recognize the need to make the changes necessary to improve the way your life will work out. On the other hand if you are reactive you more than likely blame external factors for your current situation, your genes, your lack of money, your kids your partner, etc., etc. Reactive people tend to focus on things they can't do anything about and have a habit of using terms such as "yes but...." and "if only....". They have a tendency to see the answer as outside of themselves and have reasons why it can't be done.

❧

So if we look at this with regards to losing weight we can see that the proactive response would be to take the necessary steps to ensure that you are fit and healthy or to take responsibility for your weight as soon as you realize that weight gain has become an issue. Once we let the situation get out of hand it is far more difficult to deal with.

Of course this doesn't mean you can't be proactive when you have become overweight. Taking the responsibility to be proactive and finding ways to lose the weight at any appropriate time is the best course of action.

People who are reactive regarding their weight problem will blame their genes, their metabolism, their spouse, their children, a poor education, money, etc., etc., and rather than take responsibility and do something about it, they remain overweight.

So you have a choice to be reactive and make excuses or to be proactive, take responsibility for what goes into your mouth, and make positive lasting changes.

HABIT 2: BEGIN WITH THE END IN MIND

Habit 2 requires you to use your imagination--you need to be able to envision in your mind what you cannot at present. By creating a mental image you also create a physical reality. The physical reality follows the mental, vision just as any plan on paper can be realized in the finished product.

This is an excellent visual habit for anyone who wants to be fit, healthy and slim. The law of attraction says you are what you think about. So if you think of yourselves as fat and unable to lose weight then your chances of being slim and fit and healthy are less unlikely to become a reality. However if you can envision yourself as slim and start to behave and subsequently eat like a slim person then you stand a much greater chance of this coming to fruition. If you simply live life by default then you are unlikely to achieve your dream, in this case, of being fit healthy and slim.

You need to be very clear about what it is you want. Do you want to be slim and fit and healthy? If so you have to find the determination to make the necessary changes. If you are half hearted about it then it won't happen.

Begin with the end in mind and make sure you know exactly what that is you are aiming for and when you would like to have achieved it by.

HABIT 3: PUT FIRST THINGS FIRST

Habit 3 is about life management - your purpose, values, roles, and priorities. These are the first things, the ones you prioritizeas opposed to things you say you didn't have time to do. By putting first things first, you are organizing and prioritizing your life to ensure that the long term goal you chose in habit 2 actually comes to fruition.

In the case of losing weight the first and most important thing is to ensure that you eat sensibly and understand that you are what you eat (and digest). Healthy eating becomes a priority. For example you get rid of any foods that don't help your weight loss regime and you buy only the foods that will aid your weight loss.

Many people will make the excuse that they haven't got time to prepare the food necessary for a weight loss diet. That is because they haven't given it first priority. They have seen something else as more important.

As we know many busy people manage to eat a healthy diet of real food that they cook themselves. They make that a priority over other things in their lives.

So if you truly want to eat a healthy diet and lose weight - put health first.

HABIT 4: THINK WIN-WIN

Habit 4 is about finding a solution that can benefit both sides of a dispute.

With regards to weight loss and choosing to embark on a healthy real food diet you may well be either in dispute with yourself and your feelings about this diet or you may be in dispute with your family. Families don't like change, especially if they think it is going to adversely affect them. It important therefore to persuade both yourself and your family that this is a win - win situation. If you are able to lose weight you will feel better about yourself and have more confidence and as a result your family will have a healthier and happier you. If your family is also going to be making changes to their diets because of your new regime then they need to be persuaded that they will feel healthier and be less likely to be ill in the future. You get what you want and they benefit too.

HABIT 5: SEEK FIRST TO UNDERSTAND, THEN TO BE UNDERSTOOD

Habit 5 is about communication, one of the most important skills in life.

If you're like most people, you probably seek first to be understood; you want to get your point across. And in doing so, you may ignore the other person completely, pretend that you're listening, selectively hear only certain parts of the conversation or attentively focus on only the words being said, but miss the meaning entirely.

❧❧

We are all guilty of thinking we know what is best for us and are often reluctant to listen to what others have to say. With regard to dieting we have very likely think we know what the answers are, what we need to do to lose weight. But the truth is we are still overweight and so maybe we need to listen to another person's point of view.

There is new research coming out daily regarding the best way to lose weight and sometimes it is important for us to stop and listen and not think we have all the answers. Be open to new ideas and be sure that we understand the meaning behind what we are hearing.

HABIT 6: SYNERGIZE

Habit 6 is about using synergy to your benefit. To put it simply, synergy means 'two heads are better than one'. Synergize is the habit of creative cooperation. It is teamwork, open-mindedness, and the adventure of finding new solutions to old problems. But it doesn't just happen on its own. It's a process, and through that process, people bring all their personal experience and expertise to the table. Together, they can produce far better results than they could individually. Synergy lets us discover jointly things we are much less likely to discover by ourselves. It is the idea that the whole is greater than the sum of the parts. One plus one equals three, or six. In other words it is always more than 2.

୬୬

When it comes to weight loss there are several synergistic aspects that come to mind.

Firstly there is a need for some people to lose weight by joining a group of likeminded people. Some slimming clubs however can be far too prescriptive - not allowing for creativity and diversity. Maybe also they are not recognizing the need for a different approach for different people. There is a wide range of reasons why people are overweight in the first place and this will require a wide range of approaches and understanding to help them to overcome their weight problem.

Secondly it is now possible to work with a slimming coach. The purpose of the coach will be to find an approach to changing your dietary habits that is tailor made for you.

HABIT 7: SHARPEN THE SAW

Habit 7 is about preserving the greatest asset in our lives which is ourselves. It means enhancing your ability to meet your challenges. You need to be strong in body mind and spirit. You also need to be emotionally strong. By creating this balance in our lives we are more able to deal effectively with what life throws at us.

By working on each area of your life you are working towards a balanced life, a life that is open to change and improvement.

Physical: Beneficial eating, exercising, and resting.

Social/Emotional: Making social and meaningful connections with others.

Mental: Learning, reading, writing, and teaching.

❧❧

Although the physical aspect would seem to be the one that fits most readily into the weight loss arena, in fact all four are equally relevant.

Physical - the importance of eating a healthy wholesome diet, regular purposeful exercise and adequate rest time are all vital to your weight loss success.

Social/Emotional - meeting with likeminded dieters can be a great help as can enlisting the help and support of your friends. You may want to join a slimming group in your local area or maybe an online group. It maybe that just dieting with a friend is enough to help motivate you and feel connected .

Mental - Learning about healthy eating and understanding how foods react in your body can help you to understand why you need to eat in a particular way to lose weight.

Spiritual - Meditation and relaxation can help you to be less stressed. People who are stressed are often prone to eating comfort foods. If you are relaxed and strong spiritually you are more likely to stick to your diet.

As you renew yourself in each of the four areas, you create growth and change in your life. Sharpen the Saw keeps you fresh so you can continue to practice the other six habits. You increase your capacity to produce and handle the challenges around you. Without this renewal, the body becomes weak, the mind mechanical, the emotions raw, the spirit insensitive, and the person selfish. Not a pretty picture, is it?

Losing weight doesn't just happen. Living a life in balance means taking the necessary time to renew yourself. The choice is yours, you can renew yourself through relaxation, or you can totally burn yourself out by burning the candle at both ends. You can pamper yourself mentally and spiritually, or you can go through life oblivious to your well-being. You can choose to eat healthy vibrant foods and be slim and healthy as a result or you can choose to eat sugary, processed foods and risk being unhealthy and overweight.

INDEX

❧❧

A

B

C

M

maltodextrine 7
Marc K Hellerstein 49
margarines 42
Mark Hyman MD 23
Meditation 16, 100
metabolic rate 51, 52
metabolic response 53
metabolism 16, 51, 93
Michel Montignac 55
Milk 6, 22, 54

N

nature 13, 44, 68
Nuts 70

O

Oats 22
obesity xiii, 1, 2, 9, 10, 24, 29, 32, 39, 40
obesity epidemic xiii, 1, 10
Onions 6, 23
Oranges 23
Osteoarthritis 40
oxygen 62

P

Patrick Holford 56

perpetual diet 6
photos 73, 74
Polyunsaturated fats 70
Pork 23
Potatoes 23
priorities 94
proactive 92, 93
processed foods 18, 23, 25, 101
Professor Terry Wilkins 60
purpose ii, 94, 98

R

Reactive people 92
Relaxation 16, 100, 101
resting 99
root cause 17

S

salmon 33
schools 11
seeds 70
self deception 72
selfish 100
Sharpen the Saw 99, 100
Sleep Apnea 40
Slim Fast 5
slimming clubs viii, 98
slimming coach 98

12104609R00066

Printed in Great Britain
by Amazon.co.uk, Ltd.,
Marston Gate.